20 Awesome Super Smoothies You Can't Live Without

By Kathy Tennefoss

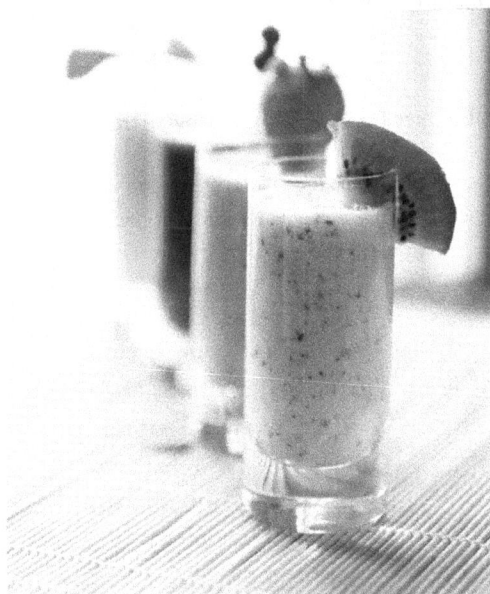

I0190597

Member of the Raw Foods Association

RECIPES 4

RAW FOOD

20 Awesome Super Smoothies You Can't Live Without

Sunny Cabana Publishing, L.L.C.

Fort Lauderdale, FL

www.sunnycabanapublishing.com

By Kathy Tennefoss

Published by Kathleen Tennefoss
Printed in the United States of America
Author: Kathy Tennefoss
Editor: Shawn M Tennefoss
13-digit ISBN: 9781936874095
10-digit ISBN: 1936874091
FIRST EDITION
Library of Congress Cataloging-in-Publication Data has been applied for

This book is dedicated to My dad James Kelley for pushing me in the right direction regarding healthy eating, living a healthy active life, and to my loving husband Shawn Tennefoss for suffering through my computer difficulties and taking the time to show me how to orchestrate this book along with sharing his life and journey with me.

Cover Design: Kathy & Shawn Tennefoss

Second Edition, 2011

Acknowledgements:

Thanks to everyone who encouraged and inspired me and gave me excellent input and feedback in the raw food industry, including one of my many sisters Heather McNerney, my husband Shawn M Tennefoss, my dad James Kelley, and Melissa Hernandez and her wonderful family! Without everyone's input I would not have finished this book or started other raw food recipe books. I am extremely grateful to everyone.
If you have any suggestions, comments, or corrections please send me an email to recipes4rawfood@yahoo.com.

Disclaimer:

The responsibility for any adverse detoxification effects resulting from using these recipes described lies not with the author or distributors of this book. This book is not intended for medical advice just as suggestion.

Please enjoy these recipes with your friends and family.

RECIPES 4

R A W   F O O D

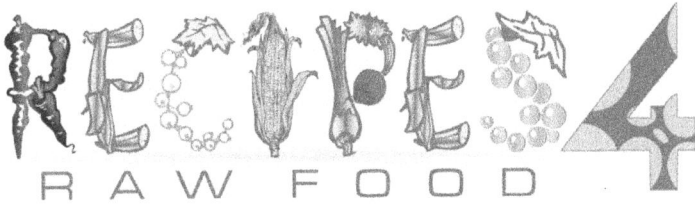

20 Awesome Super Smoothies You Can't Live Without

Raw Food Recipes for a Healthy Lifestyle

By Kathy Tennefoss

Member of the Raw Foods Association

Table of Contents

Intro

Today you hear "I'm so busy and I don't have time to eat healthy or it costs too much". Well I'm here to say that it only takes a few minutes to have a healthy meal. For the time it takes a person to go to the drive through and wait in line to have a high fat low nutrition meal you can make a quick green smoothie and head on out the door. If cost is your concern buy your organic produce in bulk or buy organic frozen fruits to add to your smoothie. You don't have to eat this way everyday but you will start to feel a difference. Your skin will start to feel better, your clothes will be fitting loser, and you might even have more energy! Isn't that worth it!

Most of these smoothie recipes are made with greens but I bet you can't even tell that they are in the smoothie. Your kids and family will be getting their greens without knowing it! They taste so good that everyone will keep asking for more! Green Smoothies are a great way to incorporate more raw greens in your diet and it is so easy!

Please try to use as much organic produce as possible when making your smoothies because when you grind up the veggies and fruits into your smoothies the produce is more concentrated. Organic produce will make the smoothies taste much better, plus you are helping the environment by purchasing organic food.

It's not necessary to use a raw food replacement powder but I tend to use it because I work out every day and it keeps me fuller. You can use other sources of protein if you like (tofu, whey, spirulina, hemp, nut butters) or not at all. Almond milk may also be substituted in the recipes for water, oat milk, hazelnut milk, etc. It's really up to your tastes buds!

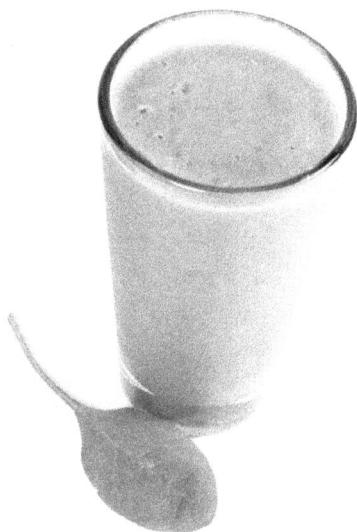

1. Popeye's Green Machine

1 Cup Almond Milk

2 Cups Spinach

$\frac{1}{4}$ Cup Aloe Vera juice

1 Scoop Raw Meal Replacement (I use Garden of Life)

1 Cup Blueberries

Splash of Lime Juice

1 Cup of ice

Mix this all in a vitamixer or blender and serve. This makes two small glasses or one large glass.

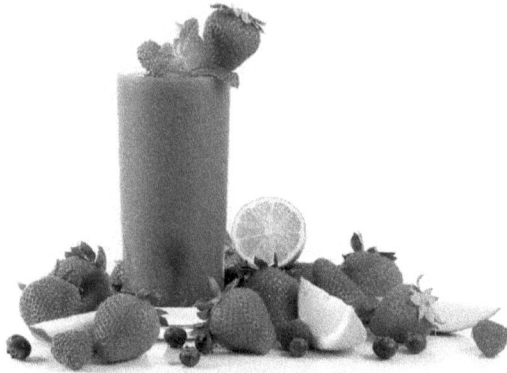

2. Strawberry Green Dream

1 Cup Almond Milk

1 Cup Spinach

1 Cup Celery

$\frac{1}{4}$ Aloe Vera juice

1 Scoop Raw Meal Replacement

1 Cup Strawberries

$\frac{1}{4}$ cup Lime Juice

1 Cup of ice

Mix all the ingredients in a vita mixer and a blender and serve. This makes two glasses or one large glass.

3. Greeneloupe

2 Cups Celery

1 Cup Almond Milk

1 Cup Cantaloupe

$\frac{1}{4}$ Cup Lime Juice

1 Scoop Raw Meal Replacement

1 Cup of ice

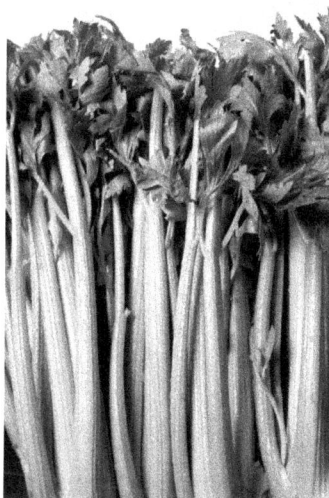

Mix all ingredients in a vita mixer or blender and serve. This makes two medium glasses.

4. What the Kale

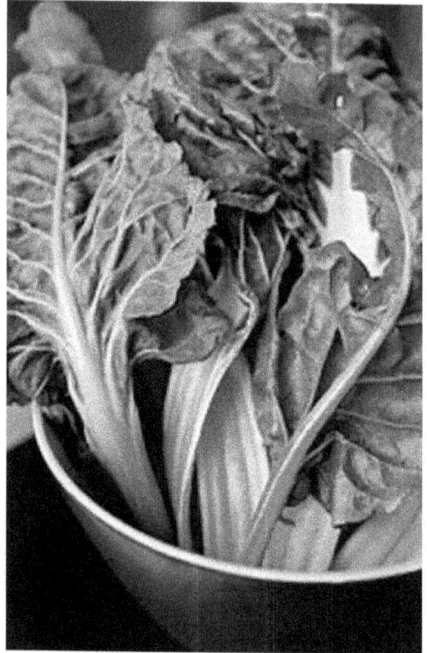

2 Cups Green Kale

1 Frozen Banana (when your bananas start to get to ripe its best to peel them and slice them in smaller pieces so that you can use them later in smoothies)

1 Cup Almond Milk

5-7 Medium Strawberries

1 Cup Blueberries

1 Scoop Raw Food Meal Replacement

1 Cup of ice

Mix ingredients in a vita mixer or blender and serve. This makes two medium glasses.

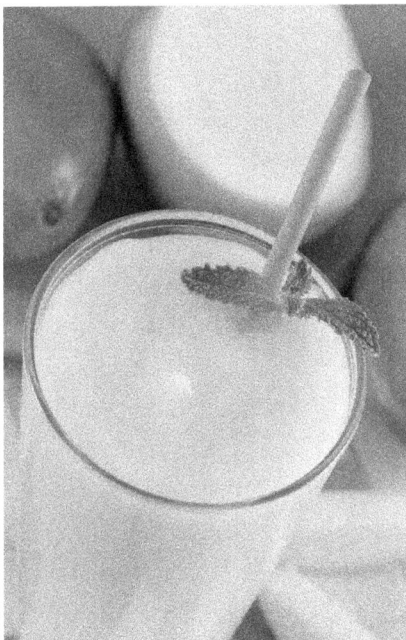

5. Mango Mamma

1 Cup Frozen Mangos (you can use fresh if you have it but the consistency will be a little thinner)

2 Cups of celery

½ Cup Almond Milk

½ Cup Orange Juice

$\frac{1}{2}$ Frozen Banana

1 Scoop of Raw Meal Replacement

1 Seeded Date

1 Tablespoon Coconut oil

1 Cup of ice

Blend all ingredients in a vita mixer or blender and serve. This makes two large glasses.

6. Acia Super Charger

1 Small Package of Frozen Acia berry (you can purchase this in most super markets or health food stores)

2 Cups Spinach

1 Cup Blueberries

$\frac{1}{2}$ Cup Almond Milk

1 Small orange peeled and cut into quarters

1 Scoop of Raw Meal Replacement

1 Cup of Ice

1 Tablespoon of Coconut oil

1 pitted date

Mix all ingredients in a vita mixer or blender and serve. This makes 2 medium glasses.

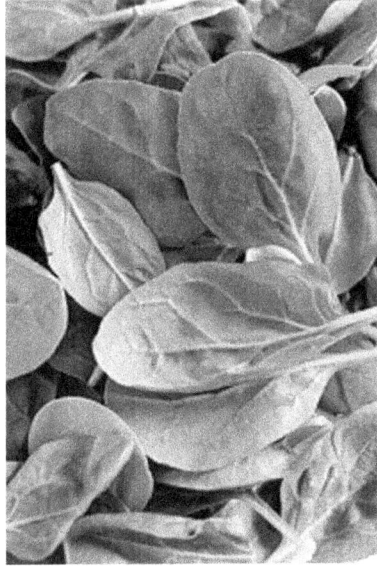

7. Peaches & Green

2 Small Peaches with the pit removed and cut into quarters

2 Cup Romaine Lettuce

1 Cup Celery

$\frac{3}{4}$ Cup of Orange Juice

1 Scoop Raw Meal Replacement

1 Cup of ice

Mix all ingredients in a vitamixer or a blender and serve. This makes two medium glasses.

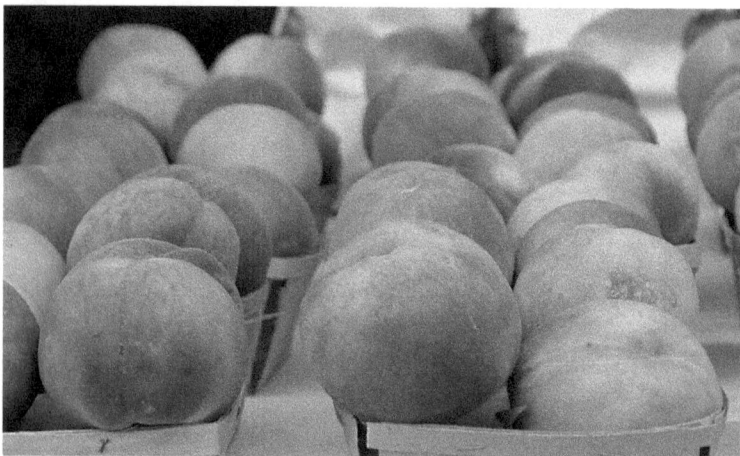

8. Green Apple

2 Cups spinach

1 Green Apple seeded and cut into quarters

¼ Cup Lime juice

1 Cup Almond Milk

1 Scoop Raw Meal
Replacement

1 Cup of ice

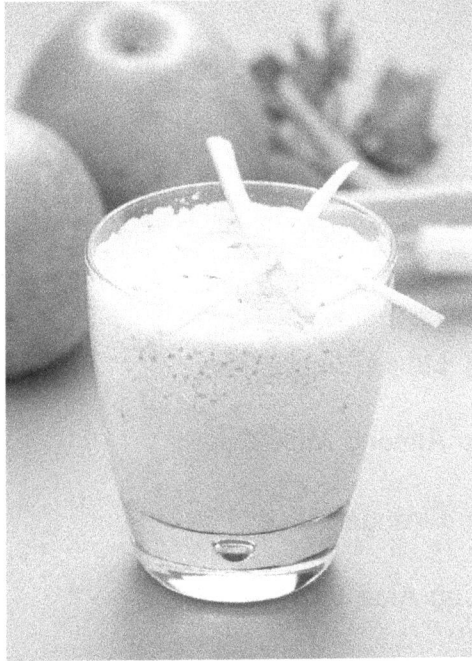

Mix all ingredients in a vita mixer or blender and serve.
This makes two small glasses.

9. Green Kiwi

1 Cup Spinach

1 Cup Celery

4 Kiwis peeled and cut

$\frac{1}{2}$ Cup Lime Juice

$\frac{1}{2}$ Cup Almond Milk

$\frac{1}{2}$ Cup Orange Juice

1/8 Cup Aloe Vera Juice

1 Scoop Raw Meal Replacement

1 Cup of ice

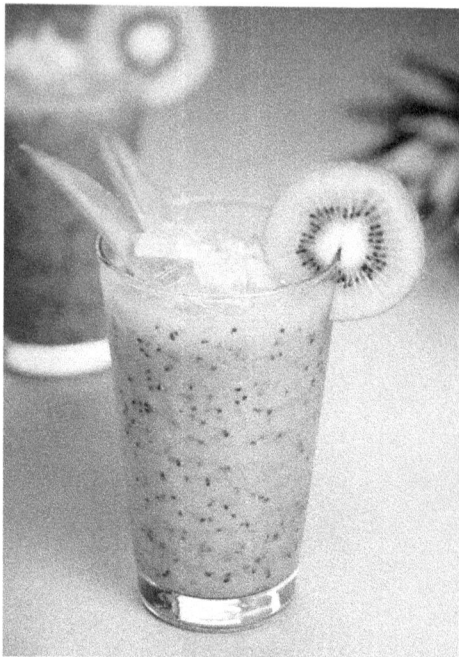

Mix all ingredients in a vita mixer or blender and serve.
This makes 2 medium glasses.

10.   Cucumber Madness

1 Large Cucumber peeled

1 Hass Avocado

$\frac{1}{4}$ Cup Lime Juice

1 Cup Water

1 Cup Ice

$\frac{1}{2}$ Bunch of Flat Leaf Parsley

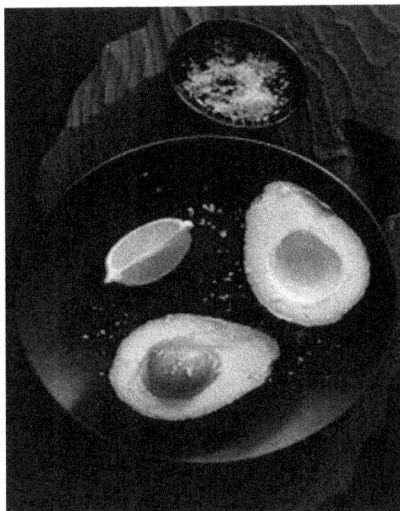

Mix all ingredients together in a vita mixer or blender and serve. This makes two small glasses.

11. Chocolate Heaven

1 Hass Avocado (pitted and sliced)

3 Tablespoons of raw cocoa powder

1 Tablespoon of agave nectar

1 Tablespoon of coconut

2 dates pitted

2 Cups Almond Milk

1 Cup of Ice

1 Frozen Banana

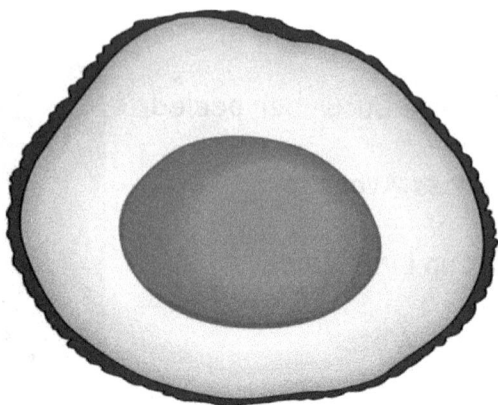

Mix all ingredients in a vita mixer or blender and serve. This is a great treat!

12.   Tropical Papaya

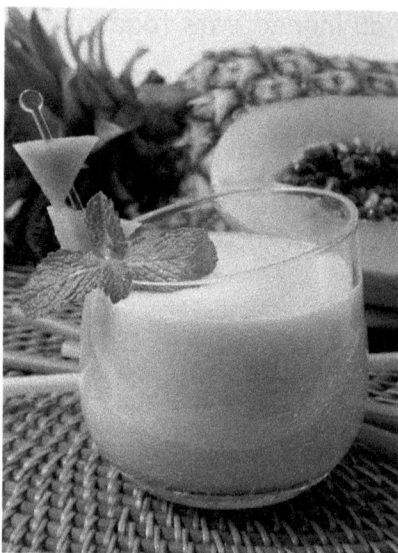

1 $\frac{1}{2}$ Cups papaya

$\frac{1}{2}$ Cup pineapple

1 Frozen Banana

1 Cup Coconut Milk

1 Cup Ice

Mix all ingredients in a vita mixer or blender and serve.
This is another yummy treat!

13.   Sweet Cherry

1 Cup Frozen Cherries

2 Cups Romaine Lettuce

1 Orange peeled and cut
into quarters

1 Cup almond milk

1 Cup Ice

Splash of Lime juice

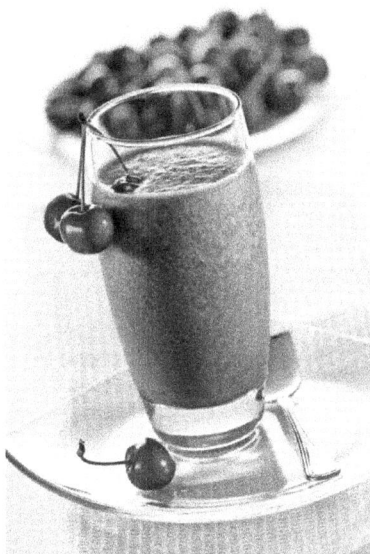

Mix all ingredients in a vita mixer or blender and serve.
This makes two small glasses.

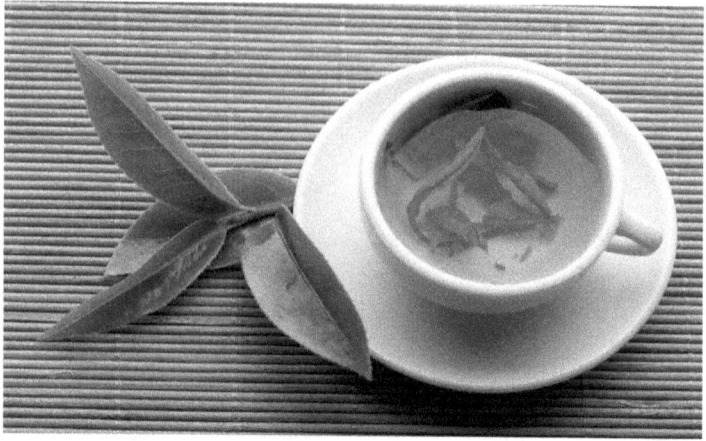

14.   Green Tea Smoothie

1 $\frac{1}{2}$ Cups of chilled green tea

1 Cup Almond Milk

1 Cup of Romaine Lettuce

1 date pitted

1 Cup of Ice

Mix all ingredients in a vitamixer or blender and serve. This is a nice and refreshing drink in the summer!

15.   Blueberry Ginger Smoothie

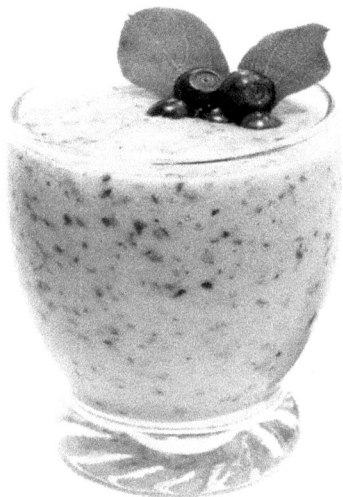

1 Cup of Blueberries

$\frac{1}{2}$ Apple (seeded and sliced)

2 Oranges peeled and sliced

1 Ginger toe peeled

$\frac{1}{2}$ Cup Almond Milk

1 Cup Romaine Lettuce or 3-4 stalks

1 Cup of Ice

Mix all ingredients in a vita mixer or a blender and serve. This makes 2 small glasses. If this is too thick you can add more almond milk or water.

16.   Pear Smoothie

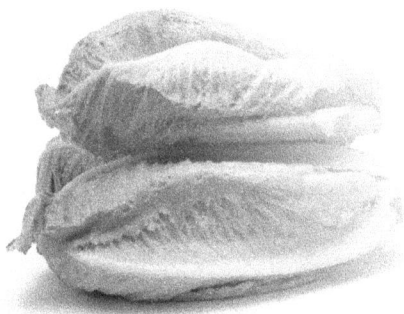

1 Pear sliced and seeded

1 Orange peeled and cut into quarters

1 Ginger Toe peeled

$\frac{1}{2}$ Frozen Banana

3-4 Stalks of Romaine Lettuce

1/2 Cup Celery

1 Cup of Almond milk

1 Cup of ice

Mix all ingredients in a vita mixer or blender and serve. This makes 2 small glasses.

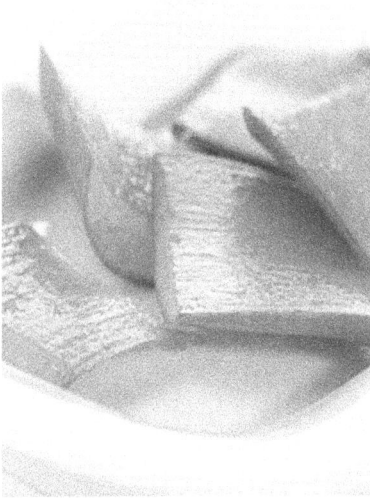

17.   Green Nectarine

5-6 Romaine Stalks

1/8 Cup of Aloe Vera Juice

1 Cup Spinach

3 Nectarines with the seed taken out

2 dates pitted

Splash of lime juice

1 Cup of ice

1 Cup of Almond Milk

Mix all ingredients in a vita mixer or blender and serve. This makes 2 small glasses.

18.   Blackberry Dream

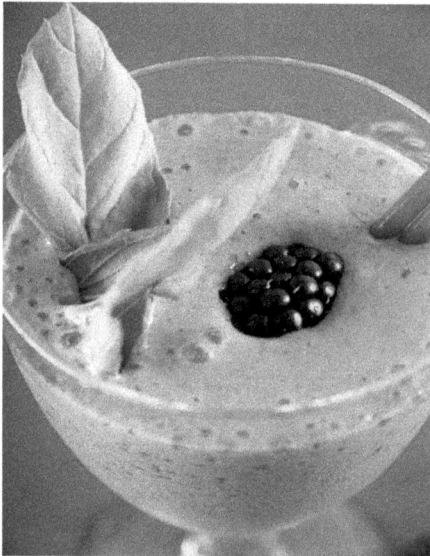

1 Raw Coconut (scoop out the inside of it)

1 Cup frozen Blackberries

2 dates pitted

4-5 Romaine Stalks

½ Frozen Banana

1 Cup Almond Milk

1 Cup of Ice

Mix all ingredients in a vita mixer or blender and serve. This makes 2 medium glasses.

19.   Mixed Green Berry

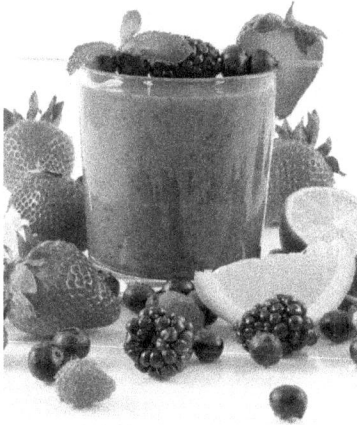

2 Cups Frozen Mixed berries

3 Cups of Spinach

½ Frozen Banana

1 Cup Almond Milk

1 Cup of Ice

1/8 Cup of Lime juice

1 Toe of ginger peeled

Mix all ingredients in a vita mixer or blender and serve. This makes two medium glasses.

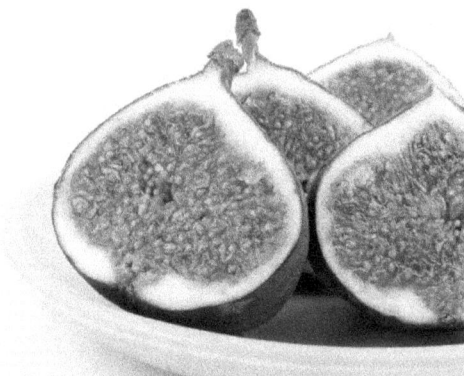

20.   Figlisious!

$\frac{1}{2}$ Cup Blueberries

3-4 Figs

1 Date pitted

2 Cups of Spinach

1 Orange peeled and quartered

1 Cup Almond milk

1 Cup of Ice

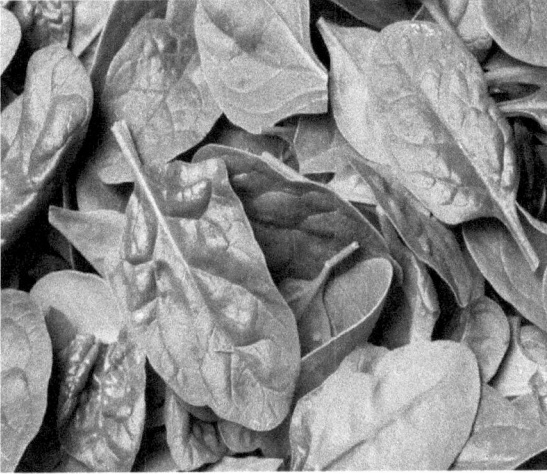

Mix all ingredients in a vita mixer or blender and serve.
This makes 2 small glasses.

I hope you enjoy my smoothie recipes! I eat them every morning and sometimes even for dinner.

You should check out some of my recipes at www.recipes4rawfood.com and www.rawfoodfortoday.com

And if you have any suggestions, comments, or corrections please feel free to email me at recipes4rawfood@yahoo.com.

I also wanted to include some very useful information on aloe vera. I use aloe vera everyday in my smoothies and I think that you will enjoy the benefits also!

The Benefits of Aloe Vera

Aloe vera was first discovered and cultivated by the Egyptians. Aloe vera grows great in a tropical environment like Florida, Hawaii, or the Caribbean.

I feel that aloe vera is one of the most beneficial plants available. Aloe vera has vitamin C, A, E and calcium, chromium, selenium, zinc, magnesium, fiber (helpful with weight loss), antioxidants, lignin's, amino acids, plant sterols (good for high cholesterol), and polysaccharides.

The benefits of aloe vera are astonishing. When you drink aloe vera juice it helps with lubricating the joints, brain, and nervous system. It is also very beneficial for the skin both internally and externally. If you tend to work out a lot or even a little then it is probably a good idea to add aloe vera juice to your diet so that your joints will last longer and function better.

Aloe vera juice also aids with digestion by giving a calming effect to the colon. It has been known to help with IBS and ulcers. I drink aloe vera juice if I have an upset stomach and it helps right away. Now the taste is something that took me a little while to get used to but now it doesn't bother me at all. Plus you can mix it in with other juices or smoothies to hide the flavor.

Aloe vera also has been shown to help with balancing out the blood sugar and lessening the symptoms of diabetics. Maybe if everyone drank aloe vera juice then we wouldn't have an epidemic of diabetes in America. It seems like everyone knows of at least one person in their life that has diabetes. So make it your quest to help others by telling them the health benefits of aloe vera juice.

It is also very beneficial for the skin both internally and externally.

Externally aloe vera is great for so many things like poison ivy or oak, rashes, acne, athlete's feet, burns, eczema, insect stings or bites, jellyfish stings, stretch marks, sunburn, varicose veins, and abrasions.

Everyone should have a bottle of organic 100% aloe vera for topical treatments and aloe vera juice to take care of the inside of your body!

About the author

B.S. Science in Physical Anthropology minor in business, and Culinary Arts Degree. Advocate for organic, vegetarian, vegan, raw food diets, writing, yoga, swimming, biking, and running 5 K's!

I have been a vegetarian/vegan/raw foodist for over 20 years. I have also worked in real estate for over ten years and have several websites to help people who are interested in raw food www.Recipes4RawFood.com and www.RawFoodForToday.com.

I have also started the Raw Foods Association with my husband so that others can become members of a larger healthy group. For more information on how to become a member the website is www.RawFoodsAssociation.com !

For more information on how to order books, original articles, become a member of the Raw Foods Association, and updates on future projects go to www.rawfoodfortoday.com or www.recipes4rawfood.com.
If you have any comments, suggestions, or corrections please feel free to email me at anytime at recipes4rawfood@yahoo.com.

Recipes 4 Raw Food
1314 E Las Olas Blvd
Fort Lauderdale, FL 33301
Recipes4rawfood@yahoo.com

www.ingramcontent.com/pod-product-compliance
Lightning Source LLC
Chambersburg PA
CBHW071801020426
42331CB00008B/2349